Disclaimer

This book is intended to be a general guide, to raise awareness, and help people make informed decisions in the context of their own personal circumstance. As everybody's circumstances are different, so are the remedies you should seek. While many of the recommendations in this book can be applied by almost anybody, regardless of their conditions, they are not intended to and should not be relied upon to replace personal medical advice.

The author accepts no responsibility for any loss or injury, be it personal or financial, as a result of the use or misuse of the information in this book. If you have any doubts or concerns after reading this book, please speak to a doctor or other qualified person before taking any action.

From The Author

Thank you for taking the time to read this book. As an author, I understand the importance of creating books which my readers will find both enjoyable and informative. If you have the time and feel generous, please don't hesitate to leave an honest review of this book.........Dr Brad Turner.

Contents

Introduction

Chapter 1

What Is Adrenal Fatigue?

Chapter 2

What Are The Signs & Symptoms Of Adrenal Fatigue?

Chapter 3

What Causes Adrenal Fatigue?

Chapter 4

Who Is Most Susceptible?

Chapter 5

Adrenal Fatigue-The Effects Of Lifestyle & Nutrition

Chapter 6

How To Determine If You Have Adrenal Fatigue

Chapter 7

How Adrenal Fatigue is Approached By Traditional Medicine

Chapter 8

Natural Methods Of Treating Adrenal Fatigue

Chapter 9

An Adrenal Fatigue Eating Plan

Chapter 10

How To Relieve Stress Naturally

Conclusion

Introduction

The human body is a combination and interconnection of various organs, which work in coordination with each other. When one part of the body fails to perform, then it hampers the rest of the body. Adrenal glands are one such important organ, which are situated on top of each of the two kidneys, and regulate the production of a lot of hormones in our body. Secretion from the two adrenal glands is important in the body, which helps store sodium. It also regulates sex hormones and maintains a glucose level in the body. This organ is very critical to the body, as it controls all the body signals, and responses with the help of the hormones it secretes. In this book we will get to know all about adrenal glands and adrenal fatigue, and also ways of combating this problem.

Chapter 1

What Is Adrenal Fatigue?

It so happens that the adrenal glands start working below its normal level and there are certain syndromes, known as signs and symptoms, which reflect the working of adrenal glands. A collection of all these signs and symptoms is known as adrenal fatigue. Mental stress is supposed to be the main cause of this kind of damage done to the body. Adrenal fatigue is also caused as a side-effect of some chronic health problems like influenza and bronchitis.

The term "fatigue" in Adrenal Fatigue is not fatigue in actual terms; rather it is more about feeling sleepy all the time, despite having proper sleep at night. The person showing symptoms of Adrenal Fatigue will act normally, and will not show some heavy signs like scars at the time of measles. The main problem with such patients is that they will not show any kind of physical illness, but internally, they will remain tired all day. Such patients tend to drink more coffee or energy boosters so that they are able to get up early in the morning and then continue with their daily course. This problem has been known with various other medical names like neurasthenia, adrenal neurasthenia and many more, and this problem is visible in a large percentage of the population in the world. There is no conventional medicine for this kind of problem and no conventional medicine has been formulated to overcome these kinds of symptoms. In short, a normal practitioner will not be able to detect this problem and tell you about it clearly. This is mainly because there is no crux theory established to determine the symptoms pointing towards adrenal fatigue.

Adrenal fatigue can cause a lot of problems in the patient's life, as the patient will not be able to leave his bed for a long period of time. The patient will need to rest in a short span of time in a day and also will not be able to undertake long duration projects. When the adrenal glands stop working further, then the body becomes weaker from inside, and body organs will suffer in the process. A lot of negative changes happen when adrenal glands do not work properly. Your carbohydrate, protein, vitamins and metabolism stop working properly. The cardiovascular system, in the long run, stops working normally. Eventually, even the sex drive in the body is affected. All the other systems of body actually change their functioning so that they are able to support the vacuum created by the non-functioning of the adrenal glands. Over time, other parts of the body are not able to take the pressure of non-functional adrenal glands. Many changes take place inside the body, so that the body is able to carry on its day to day activities, but when the adrenal glands' function is stopped permanently, it then becomes impossible for the body to work properly.

Chapter 2

What Are The Signs & Symptoms Of Adrenal Fatigue?

We will discuss the signs, which a person feels and even the signs which others can see in a patient. These signals and signs inform you about your ill health. There is a major difference between a sign and a symptom. Symptoms are felt from the external to your inner self and only you are able to understand such symptoms; for example, feeling constant pain in your head. Signs are visible to other people. They are able to detect such signs, and inform you that something is wrong with you; for example, some kind of skin rash. It is always important to collect all such signs and symptoms about your ill health and take precautionary measures well in advance. In this chapter, we will see all such signs and symptoms separately.

SYMPTOMS

Hair Loss: If you are losing a lot of hair, despite normal weather conditions, then you should note this situation and get yourself checked for any kind of hormonal imbalance in your body.

Excess sweet and salt craving: Normally, you do not eat sweets, but all of a sudden you feel like eating a lot of chocolates, etc... This is not a normal situation and you should take it seriously.

Tiredness: If you are taking a full 6-8 hours of sound sleep at night on a daily basis, but still you do not feel like waking up in the morning or you feel sleepy for the whole day, then you should get yourself checked. This is not a normal physical condition. You can also feel some body aches when you wake up in the morning, or during the day.

Energy imbalance: Sometimes, it may happen that you feel energized in the afternoon rather than in the morning and this is a signal of the onset of adrenal fatigue. This happens due to the fact that damage control process of adrenal glands start working only after the day starts, when you drain out on natural energy. To maintain energy throughout the day, you might also feel like having a coffee or any kind of energy stimulant. If you feel a surge in craving for coffee, then it is time to watch out.

Weight Loss: If you belong to the group of "healthy", then this symptom will definitely not go unnoticed. If you feel that you have lost unnecessary weight, without putting in much effort, then this should worry you.

SIGNS

Hollow Cheeks: This happens when the adrenal glands are non-functioning, and the patient tends to eat more sugar and carbohydrates. The patient should check his diet immediately and then combat the situation in time.

Lines on fingertips: This is one easy sign, which can be detected by anyone around you. You look at your fingertips and see whether they are plump and soft or they are rough and full of vertical lines. If your fingers have vertical lines, then for sure you are suffering from some kind of adrenal stress and you should have a checkup done.

Pale Lips: Check the color of your lips. Are they pink or are they pale looking? If your lips are pale looking then that might not be a sign of aging, but you might be suffering from some kind of stress or irregular dietary habits.

Muscle Pain: Muscle pain is one sign which defines adrenal problems accurately. You will feel pain in knees and back muscles without you having done any kind of physical labor. You must definitely look for such signs and take necessary measurements.

Chapter 3

What Causes Adrenal Fatigue?

Adrenal fatigue is a problem which affects all age groups. It can generally be felt and experienced by anyone and at any point in time. For example, the general physical dullness experienced at the time of some emotional trauma, financial crisis or some other kind of personal crisis. You will be amazed to know that adrenal fatigue will still hit the person, even when he has good food, takes proper sleep and lives in a stress free environment. When the problem is so grave, you are advised to establish the reasons or the causes of such a grave problem. But it is noteworthy to mention that the causes are related to slow- or non-working adrenal glands, which then leads to adrenal fatigue. We will discuss this in detail below.

Illness or Disease: Diseases and illnesses are the major causes of slow working adrenal glands. The diseases can be as minor as flu and skin allergy as well as some kind of grave diseases like bronchitis, pneumonia and etc. When a person suffers from such disease, the adrenal glands are supposed to produce required hormones that will address the internal damage caused due to the illness. Now, if the adrenal gland stops functioning properly during illness, then the patient suffers from adrenal fatigue.

Exposed to Toxic Chemicals: Let us assume, hypothetically, that you are working in some kind of chemical manufacturing company. You will be handling various chemicals. Some of these chemicals can be very harmful to your body. Now, this is a bad environmental condition for your body, and important hormones in your body will not work properly. In such cases, adrenal glands will increase the production of hormones, which will balance out the slow working of other hormones in your body. Consequently, it will stop functioning properly after some time. Once the adrenal glands break down, your body will suffer from adrenal fatigue.

Physical Surgery: Once again, let us take an example and try and understand this condition. Suppose a person has undergone some kind of leg surgery. Then, a great deal of hormones is secreted in order to recover from that surgery. In this process, a lot of stress is born by the adrenal glands. If the surgery is not cured for a long time, then adrenal glands face a lot of pressure from secreting excessive hormones. Over time, excess stimulation of glands results in slow functioning of adrenal glands, which results in symptoms related to adrenal fatigue.

Personal Problems Or Financial Issues: The work of the adrenal glands is to mobilize every response in the body, to any kind of stressful situation in life, be it emotional or physical. Adrenal glands produce the required hormones responsible for the production of energy for the body. This process is also known as homeostasis. Now, if this particular process slows down, then a person can feel adrenal fatigue. Again, if the adrenal gland is overburdened with the trauma for a longer duration of time, then it will stop working properly and the person will undergo symptoms of adrenal fatigue. If a person gets worried about small issues, then he will feel stressed even in inconsequential matters. The person facing excessive stress will also face adrenal fatigue often, as compared to the person who tackles all kinds of negative situations relatively calmly.

Chapter 4

Who Is Most Susceptible?

People, who suffer from Adrenal Fatigue, are highly susceptible to various kinds of dangers in life. If you are the one suffering from adrenal fatigue, then you will be prone to other damages happening to your body. Adrenal Fatigue is the term given to that stage, wherein the adrenal glands are overloaded with the secretion of hormones in the body and they start to underperform. If you are suffering from adrenal fatigue, it means your body is not producing necessary hormones in adequate amounts, and also all the body organs are not able to function properly. The hormones secreted by adrenal glands control all the organ functions of the body. If the adrenal glands stop working, then it is very dangerous.

In the short run, you feel tired and will not be able to cope with the pressures and demands of life. However, this pressure will not show up physically in your body. It is in the later stage of adrenal gland failure that you will be able to feel that your many body organs have stopped working properly, which is bad news. You will find that your thyroid glands have stopped secreting thyroxin and you are not able to carry on your bodily functions properly.

Chapter 5

Adrenal Fatigue-The Effects Of Lifestyle & Nutrition

Earlier in this book, we discussed the various factors leading to adrenal fatigue in a person's life. However, if you examine the facts minutely, then you will realize that all the causes and reasons broadly fall, some way or another, in the category of an unhealthy lifestyle. This unhealthy lifestyle also consists of unhealthy eating habits, which we were developed recently. If you really want to ensure that your adrenal glands work properly, then you should first look into the kind of lifestyle you are living and try to change the negative aspects of this lifestyle.

Lifestyle

Lifestyle may be just one word, but connotes a lot of meaning. Lifestyle is basically the way you conduct your life, and what your daily routine is in life. This particular daily routine affects you both mentally as well as physically, and thus, it is important to determine the constituents of an unhealthy lifestyle; that lifestyle which leads to adrenal fatigue.

Sleeping Time: Doctors advise that a person should go to sleep at 11PM and take at least 6 hours of sound sleep. During this time, the body hormones cleanse themselves and if we remain awake during this time, then our body will be full of toxic material. Nowadays, people stay up really late due to cell phones and other devices. This is a major reason for the rampant growth of adrenal fatigue among the younger generation.

Living a Stressful Life: People have gotten used to taking a lot of tension in their lives, right from their childhood. They strive for each and every thing in their life, and actually build up a lot of pressure and tension, just to cope with their own set of expectations. This particular lifestyle, wherein taking tension and then completing the work has become a style statement, hampers the adrenal glands of a person. Rather than worrying so much about small issues of life, it is important to live life tension free, but it seems that this is one fact not known to many people.

Nutrition

Nutrition and dietary habits are another factor which affects how the adrenal glands work.

Excess of Carbohydrates: If you have a habit of eating more carbohydrates rather than proteins, then it puts a lot of unnecessary pressure on adrenal glands to digest those carbohydrates. Carbohydrates break into sugar molecules in the body, which is the actual damaging content for adrenal glands. Nowadays, more and more people have gotten used to having a lot of sugar in their coffee, aerated drinks, and fast food. This is very harmful for the body. There is also one phenomenon of taking fewer proteins in the diet which adds on to the gravity of the problem. If you are able to watch your diet, you will be able to perform better.

Maintain Eating Schedule: It is always advised to maintain a proper schedule for eating, especially if you are already suffering from adrenal fatigue. At this time, the body is not able to maintain a proper balance of body salt and thus, you must never skip a meal while you are suffering from adrenal fatigue. You should eat small meals every two hours, and the food should be rich in good cholesterol, proteins and adequate amounts of carbohydrates. This will ensure that you do not suffer from adrenal fatigue because of nutritional deficiencies.

Chapter 6

How To Determine If You Have Adrenal Fatigue

Adrenal fatigue or adrenal exhaustion shows some common body changes and it affects many aspects of our life. It is not simple to determine adrenal fatigue by taking one or two factors into consideration. The following are the most popular methods of diagnosis that have been practiced all over the world:

History & Questionnaire

Medical history of symptoms and a medically formed questionnaire is being designed especially to rule out adrenal fatigue. It covers all the stress related symptoms and other medically important signs. Although the questionnaire is not the only diagnostic method, at least it makes the picture clear and gives doctors an easy time in conducting further tests to determine the condition.

It is a scale based test in which patients are asked to rate a number of questions from 0 to 3. The rating is divided into two parts, with the patient asked to rate the same question with relevance to past experience and also present experience.

Scaling method
0 indicates never happened
1 indicates occasionally happened

2 indicates moderate intensity/frequency

3 indicates severe/intense frequency

Sample Questionnaire

The total questionnaire is divided into multiple parts. It covers sections like predisposing factors, key signs and symptoms, frequent events, pattern of energy level, aggravating elements, diet or food pattern and relieving factors. Some of the questions are as follows:

- •I feel better after a stressful situation is resolved.

- •I crave foods high in salt more frequently. I like salty foods more.

- •I frequently get rashes and dermatitis.

- •I have experienced severely stressful events which affect my well being.

- •I had recurring and intense respiratory infections.

- •I am suffering from frequent nervous stomach indigestion at stressful times.

- •My sex drive has been affected and has reduced.

- •I feel much better most of the time. After a noon meal I feel fully awake.

- •My thinking has become confused at times when I am in a hurry or feel under pressure.

Saliva Testing

Our adrenal glands secrete hormones which are the main culprits behind our response to stress. The rise and fall of the adrenal hormone called "Cortisol" tells the whole story of the fluctuation of stress response. Cortisol levels are the most trusted factor in determining the functionality of adrenal glands. The cortisol test of saliva is carried out to measure the level of cortisol and another critical hormone called DHEAS.

The test is carried out to understand the extent of hormonal imbalance; it becomes extremely important to reveal underlying causing factors like anxiety, obesity, depression, diabetes etc. In the test, the patient is asked to spit into the test tube multiple times during the day. Each time, the patient's sputum is analyzed to determine the level of cortisol in it. A total of four times the sample is being tested; first sample is taken at 8 AM and then it is subsequently tested at noon, 4 PM and at midnight. Not only cortisol, but other steroid hormones are also taken into consideration like testosterone, progesterone etc. The World Health Organization (WHO) has confirmed the accuracy of the saliva test in determining adrenal fatigue.

Pupillary Response Test

This is not a medical test carried out at a medical center; rather it is one of the determining methods that people can carry out in their home. Here are the steps to carry out the test:

•For at least 10 to 15 minutes, continuously stand in front of a mirror. Be sure that the room is darkened; the best time to carry this out is after sunset.

•Now, without blinking, look straight and with the help of a flashlight/penlight. Hold the head at least 8 inches away and in a manner that it points to your ear. The 8 inch distance is kept to protect the eye.

•Be careful that the light does not reflect directly into your retinas. You should not feel like a "deer in headlights". Stop at the point when the light reflects at a 45 degree angle to your retina.

•Hold the seconds up to which you can stand without blinking. In normal condition, an individual can stand more than 20 seconds.

Indications:

0 – 4 seconds – Suggestive of Adrenal Exhaustion

5 – 10 seconds – Suggestive of Adrenal Fatigue

11 – 19 seconds – Suggestive of Adrenal Dysfunction

Chapter 7

How Adrenal Fatigue is Approached By Traditional Medicine

Adrenal fatigue can be approached by two popular treatment methods. One is through medication involving standard medicine that is prescribed by a specialist doctor and another involving Traditional Chinese Medicine (TCM). Apart from these two traditional methods of treatment, one can also cure it naturally, which we will cover in the next chapter.

Commonly Practiced Medicicines

Considering the medical history over time, there are few medicines that have been used to treat adrenal fatigue. A particular drug may not be used in treatment in a particular country; treatment course may differ from county to country. Please do not take these medicines on your own, kindly consult a doctor for a prescription.

List of some of the common drugs prescribed:

•Solu-Medrol Injection

•Dexamethasone Intensol

•Methylprednisolone Sodium Succinate Intravenous

•Hydrocortisone Sodium Succinate Injection

•Hydrocortisone Sodium Succinate (PF) Injection

•Dexamethasone Sodium Phosphate Injection

•Depo-Medrol Injection

•Betamethasone Acet & Sodium Phosphate Injection

Traditional Chinese Medicinal Treatment

Chinese medicinal approach for the treatment of adrenal fatigue is more focused on the energy and chemistry. On the other hand, occupational medicines are more focused on treating hormonal changes. In the Chinese method, the energy generated from the adrenal part of the kidney is called "Kidney Chi". It is believed that the Kidney Chi is given to the individual during birth time and it is responsible for cell growth and cell division. It acts as a life force.

The same energy is responsible for sexual potency, fertility and physical endurance. Chinese tradition believes that the vital energy can be restored with the help of Chinese herbal medicines, Acupuncture, Deep relaxation technique, Emotional Balancing technique and Taoist breathing exercises.

Acupuncture is directed towards regaining optimal health and full body energy by restoring the baseline over time. Numerous health programs are being conducted every year that focus on how to de-stress the surrounding environment. Other traditional Chinese methods have become a popular choice of treatment as they teach the importance of resting, as well as a peaceful and calm mind to treat millions of individuals suffering from adrenal fatigue.

This traditional method sheds light on the role of inner fire and spirit to restore the function of deficient kidneys. The method of treatment surrounds and replenishes kidneys so that the fire and inner peace can reach to the heart for one's well being. The treatment is carried out with the help of various herbal formulas mentioned below:

- Achyranthes & Rehmannia Formula

- Lycium Formula

- Anemarrhena formula

- Phellodendron and Rehmannia Formula

- Combined Ginseng Nutritive Formula

- Combined Astragalus & Pueraria Formula

- Tortoise Shell Formula

- Eucommia Formula

- Deer Antler

- Deer Horn Formula

Patients are advised to take a certain combination of formulas 3 times a day with warm water. It helps in regaining the tone of the kidney by nourishing it from inside. Different formulas are aimed at notifying blood and warming the kidney to promote water movement.

Chapter 8

Natural Methods Of Treating Adrenal Fatigue

Along with medicinal methods for treatment, it is very important to follow natural methods as they are easy to practice at home and can control adrenal fatigue. It helps in diminishing and relieving signs and symptoms.

Naturally Energizing Electrolyte

Foods that contain high amounts of electrolyte substances have been proven medically to keep adrenal fatigue symptoms at bay. Add them in your regular intake of water or meals to ensure you get a sufficient amount of electrolyte in a single day; they contain the positive charge that helps in regulating muscle functions, maintaining acid-base balance and keeping fluid balance intact in the body. Lemon, pork, beef, olives, etc. are some electrolyte rich foods. A daily supply of 23000 mg is sufficient to keep cortisol under warning level.

Apply Raw Oats As A Nerve Tonic

Avena sativa is another common food that can be used instead of raw oats. Although it is a food type, we are not referring to it as a food, but very few people know about its beneficial effect on nerves. That is why it is medically known as an herbal element. In can also be wrapped in a cheesecloth sack with jasmine and added in a bath to soothe your skin.

Time Your Meals And Snacks

Lack of food intake for long periods stimulates the kidneys to release more cortisol and adrenal hormones, which disturbs proper bodily functions. Even at the time of sleeping, our body remains in need of energy. Without proper sugar levels, our body triggers a stress reaction which puts pressure on adrenal glands. Timely eating allows regulation of cortisol level.

Cortisol levels take the root of natural circadian rhythm. It starts to increase around 6 am and reaches optimal level around 8 am. During the day time, it falls and rises again as per body needs. Proper timing maintains the natural route of cortisol. It is advised to eat larger meals at the beginning of the day to support cortisol level throughout the day. One should also eat smaller meals during the day to keep the cortisol level in check.

Treat Yourself With Chamomile

This is one method unknown to many. However, it has worked for many adrenal fatigue patients. One can create chamomile lawn around his house. Its magical aroma lightens the mood and calms the nerves. It reduces the nerve activity and makes you relax. Put 3-4 cups of chamomile flowers in your bath, lie down, and enjoy the natural aroma.

Avoid Stimulants

Drinks and beverages that are high in stimulants must be avoided. Adrenal fatigue symptoms can trigger with high consumption of caffeinated and caloric drinks. We will discuss more about the diet control plan later in this book.

Implement A Light Evening Diet

The secret to a peaceful and cozy night sleep pattern lies in the evening diet. It is very important to follow this as it can rejuvenate the body in the morning and supply you with much needed energy levels. Passiflora incarnate is the fusion drink than is made from passion flower and chamomile. Drink a cup of the fusion to get rid of lazy mornings.

Tackle The Stress Demon

Keeping stress under control resolves half of the problems and symptoms that trouble you. Ancient stress relieving techniques like meditation, yoga, tai chi etc. have helped millions of people to get over negative effects of stress. Later in this book we will cover natural techniques in details to tackle stress.

Chapter 9

An Adrenal Fatigue Eating Plan

It has been proven that diet has significant role to play in curing adrenal fatigue. It starts from selecting the food you eat, managing the schedule and goes on. Follow these simple steps to manage fatigue.

Manage Your Diet- Choose The Right Foods

Increasing the levels of vitamin C and B5 in the diet has helped in easing adrenal fatigue symptoms. Foods like red bell peppers, papaya, citrus and broccoli are rich sources of vitamin C; similarly yogurt, sunflower seeds, mushrooms, and corn have vitamin B5 in great amounts.

Too much caffeine intake also stimulates cortisol production. To curb the intake of caffeine, you can gradually replace soda and coffee with low-caffeine beverages. Green tea is a great substitute.

It is natural to have a craving for sweets when there is low blood sugar in the body. But one must control the intake of a diet that can worsen the condition. Food items that must be avoided for frequent consumption are cookies, candy, colas, coffee drinks, doughnuts, and other tasty snacks. The energy is short lasting that has been derived from these types of food. Both stress and exhaustion along with hunger dampen our ability for make the right choice of food. One must remind himself about the negative side effects of eating food that is in the danger zone; with patience and control one can overcome his own strong desire for these foods. Refined carbohydrates and caffeine products unknowingly puts us at risk of greater health hazard by disturbing sleep patterns and body function that only worsens the fatigue symptoms.

Coffee Substitutes

Individuals with a strong desire to beat adrenal fatigue have many options that can replace coffee intake. Green tea with roasted rice is popularly called "Genmaicha", it contains a very small amount of caffeine with roasted and rich flavor. Additionally nuts, grains, herbs, and various fruits can be roasted same as coffee to get real coffee like flavor. Some of the favorite ones are barley, chicory root, and dandelion root.

Roastaroma: A tea blend made from roasted barley, roasted carob and roasted chicory root. Additionally, spices are added like cinnamon.

Genmaicha: A type of green tea along with roasted brown rice. The green tea has nutty and mellow flavor.

Teechino: Made from the fusion of roasted chicory, carob, and, roasted barley. For sweetness and nutty flavor, almonds and dates are added. It is available in different blends of flavors like hazelnut, java, vanilla etc.

Cafix: Made from chicory and barley, it is freeze dried to make it available in powder and crystal form. It contains 0% caffeine.

Pero: Originating from Switzerland, Pero is made from mixing barley, rye and chicory in certain amounts.

Plan It Out – Maintain A Proper Diet Schedule

To lessen the effect of high levels of cortisol, one must make a firm and workable diet plan to practice and follow routinely in their life. The more you become strict about your diet plan, the less the likelihood to opt for medicinal approach.

- Get up and eat breakfast within an hour, 8 am at the latest. It restores blood sugar levels that have decreased during night time.

- Before 9 am, eat a healthy snack.

- Take lunch between 11-12 am. It prevents a large dip in the amount of cortisol in the body.

- Consume a healthy snack in the duration between 2 and 3 pm as this is the time when cortisol levels begin to drop significantly. Do not make a mistake by consuming caffeinated drinks.

- Make dinner time around 6-7 pm; it is very hard to eat that early, but eat a light meal in the starting days. With time you will used to it.

- Before going to sleep, eat light snacks at least one hour earlier. It will protect you from dropping sugar level during sleep.

Ways To Eat To Support Adrenal Health

Our day to day eating habits also contribute to our condition; be attentive while purchasing the food you eat. Minor things can go unnoticed and then make it very difficult to control adrenal hormones. Follow these tips to get healthy habits to keep adrenal functions going normally.

- •Consume more organic, seasonal, wholesome and locally grown foods.

- •Foods with artificial color, preservatives, dyes and added hormones must be avoided.

- •Lean protein is a great source that helps in stabilizing sugar level. Include these foods in the list.

- •Purchase foods from health stores that give you natural and whole food items.

Chapter 10

How To Relieve Stress Naturally

Stress is the bug which requires the utmost concentration and state of mind to deal with. Do not allow this bad bug to disturb your thought process and lifestyle; kick it out with some natural remedies. Some of the best relaxation methods have been explored in this chapter for living stress free life.

The Importance Off The Biological Cycle

Our body hormones like cortisol control our various body functions including our thinking pattern. Your moods and behavior depend on the amount of the hormones present in the body. If normal secretion gets disturbed, it negatively affects our thinking process.

Routine works and pattern include
- Sleep pattern and duration of sleep as in number of hours.

- Type of diet taken on a regular basis.

- Working hours and pleasure time for relaxation.

Sunlight therapy
The effect of light is something ignored by many. You must note that sunlight is also an excellent alternative and natural way to cure stress. Sunlight works as clock setter for the mind; that is why the internal clock, also called the biological clock, sets its time based on sunlight exposure. If

the clock gets disturbed, it affects body energy level, appetite, sleep etc.

Many people experience a cyclic intense stress period during the short and dark days of winter season. This is commonly referred to as seasonal affective disorder. That is why exposure to at least half an hour to sunlight is necessary to avoid negative thoughts and altered life pattern. Ideally, as much as 1 to 2 hours of daily exposure is considered to be beneficial.

Get control over negative thoughts

The battle of stress management is best managed by the mind. It is how our mind thinks that makes or breaks things. Our state of stress has the most common link with negative thought processes. Often in the state of depression, people think with the mind set of worst possible scenarios. Challenging the negative thought process is the natural way to cure common sadness.

Of course it is not easy to think positively overnight and change one's mindset completely. But with focus and right attitude, it will start to affect you positively in order to reduce the effect of stress. One effective way is to list all your problems on paper. Problems seem bigger in the mind, but when you start applying thought to it, problems do not appear as serious as we thought. Avoid focusing on problems that are completely unnecessarily troubling you. Positive mindset increases serotonin level in the body to keep a happy mood. Popularly used meditation techniques help in increasing dopamine levels that also work on the same logic as serotonin.

Yoga Therapy

It has been well known all around the world about the effects of the ancient Indian Yoga techniques. Yoga is believed to dampen the effect of stress causing substances and aids in relaxing the state of mind. According to reports, Yoga affects more in relieving symptoms of stress than any other type of exercises.

Following is a list of some of the most popular Yoga positions to manage stress:

Adho Mukha Svanasana: This position helps in bringing back one's energy level and fights back anxiety level.

Paschimottanasana: This position helps in fighting depression by making one more alive, and gives relief from despondency.

Prasarita Padottanasana: This position helps in reduction of fatigue level and soothes out jittery nerves.

Dwi Pada Viparita Dandasana: This position helps in invigorating the body and lifting up the spirit.

Urdhva Dhanurasana: This position helps in improving blood circulation, creates feelings of well being and stimulates the nervous system.

Balasana: This position helps in decreasing irritability symptoms, balances the emotions and balances the functions of the endocrine system.

Relaxation Response Technique

Relaxation technique works on the principle that is opposite of stress. With mastering, this technique one can manage high blood pressure and anxiety level. It slows down breathing patterns by 25 percent and consumption of oxygen gets lowered by 17 percent. It flushes out negative thoughts and significantly reduces stress related side effects.

- Select a quite place and sit comfortably. Now relax your muscles gradually and close your eyes.

- Choose your favorite word, a prayer that enlightens you the most. You must have firm belief in the word to make you peaceful. The purpose is to minimize your mind activity.

- Take repeated breathing session by inhaling through nose and exhaling though mouth. Maintain focus on the word or prayer. Keep repeating it along with maintaining breathing session.

- Just try to lose focus on the present issues troubling you. Stop thinking about it and dislodge the thought that makes you negative. It might be difficult, but with time you will be able to improve focus. Sit quietly and explore the new state of peace and inner calm.

Practice this for about 20-25 minutes regularly and repeat twice or thrice a week. There is no fixed timing although, one can do sessions for as long as one enjoys and can keep the focus intact.

Stess Releaving Exercises

Exercises are the best when it comes to stress management. Some specific sets of exercise benefit a lot by giving strength to fight stress causing elements and keep a calm mind. It improves the body's capacity to deal with stress and negative thoughts.

Deep Breathing Exercises

One can take sessions of these exercises without any particular time frame. It is more practical in nature and involves diaphragmatic movement shifts to practice and master it. Quick and shallow breathing stimulates the stress causing factors which makes a person uncomfortable and causes anxiety. Deep breathing eliminates stress and generates the body's natural response.

Muscle Relaxation Exercises

Our body experiences tension in the muscles during states of stress or anxiety. It is a progressive technique to relax muscles. This muscular technique energizes the body by reducing muscle tension to save energy. Commonly, the exercises are practiced in a comfortable chair.

Conclusion

Adrenal fatigue does not look like a grave body situation, but its underlying post effects are very harmful for the body. Adrenal fatigue is a kind of signal that the body gives you, when your body is not functioning properly, and you should be wise enough to catch those signals. If you are able to detect the problem early, then you will save yourself from all the major problems that arise after the non-functioning of adrenal glands.

In this book, we have seen various figments related to adrenal fatigue. We have gotten to know about the basics of adrenal fatigue, its causes, symptoms, and cure. This book is the perfect guide to a good life, if you learn and follow the guidelines set herein.

Other Books By Dr Brad Turner

Headache Cures Made Easy

Headaches are extremely common, especially in today's society where everyone is stressed, exhausted and forever taking on too much work. However, the big problem arises when we stop viewing headaches as something serious. Whether large or small, headaches can often be a symptom of a more severe underlying problem and ignoring them is the worst thing we can do. Whether you regularly experience primary or secondary headaches, you can use this 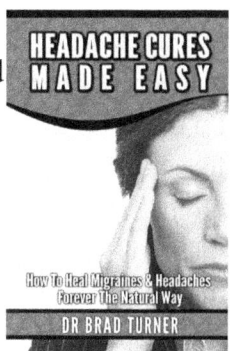 guide to learn about the causes of headaches, the symptoms that can arise and how to tackle them if they are a common occurrence in your life. It also offers you details of natural cures, giving you useful tips and ideas to help stop that headache in its tracks, as well as information on how to prevent getting headaches and migraines in the future.

Lose Belly Fat Without Exercise

Dr Brad Turner's *Lose Belly Fat Without Exercise is* an easy to follow guide which gives you the important information you need to give you a jump start to a vibrant, radiant and sexy new you!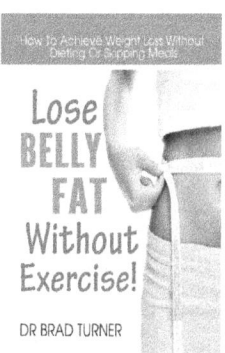

If you are tired of counting calories, fat grams and points and or have lost your motivation with crash course Exercise programs and are tired of diets that just do not work, then this book is for you.

.

Aromatherapy The Beginner's Guide

Frankincense. Peppermint. Eucalyptus. Lemon-grass. Lavender. Who knew that these are five of the must have essential oils? Dr. Brad Turner does—and we are blessed that he's chosen to share his knowledge and expertise in his latest book, ESSENTIAL OILS. So much has been written about using oils: as cures for everything from toothaches to acne; aromatherapy and even taken internally for whatever reason is popular that day. To our own peril, we've discovered much of this information is false. Dr. Turner gains our trust immediately with his treatise: never ingest these essential oils. And that's the beginning of an author/reader relationship that will stand the test of time…and information, because Dr. Turner tells the truth. And that's the way we like it!

The Type 2 Diabetes Cure

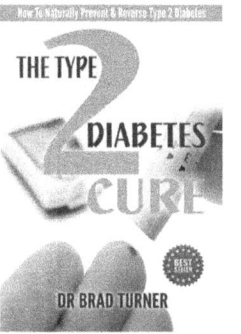

TYPE 2 DIABETES CURE just blew the myths out of the water concerning diabetes. It's the ultimate guide to diabetes, no matter the type. By defining all three types of diabetes, the author helps readers understand just how easy it is to overcome type 2 diabetes. From the sampling of mouth-watering recipes to eating plans, to exercise recommendations —TYPE 2 DIABETES CURE tells the truth--type 2 diabetes can be cured as well as prevented. And, that, my friends, is the most wonderful message in the book! Get your copy today and start your journey to incredible health.

Quit Smoking Naturally

On every literary corner, there's an expert on how to quit smoking. But very few of their theories stick. Every day the weary smoker is inspired to quit, only to have his/her hopes dashed yet again. Quit Smoking Naturally is the book that may set everyone free! The genius of this book is the straightforward approach and authentic voice that provides the facts, dispels the fallacies and motivates the smoker to do what they've never done before—succeed at quitting!

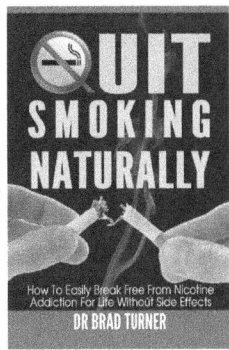

Natural Antibiotics And Antivirals For Beginners

Herbs are among the first providers of medicines that had been used by our ancestors thousands of years ago. Since then, the world has developed sufficiently and new medicines made of various chemicals have been introduced to the people. However, this does not lessen the effective medicinal properties of the herbs. If anything, they can still be the most convenient sources of medicines.

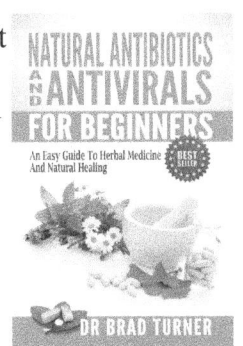

This book is a record of the various medical herbs and their properties. It also entails the preparations of the medicines from these herbs. Herbal medicines have the capacity of curing infections and diseases in the most convenient way. Not only that, but they are also almost completely harmless and have no side-effects whatsoever. The need for such medicines has become very intense since our bodies have developed a capacity to get used to the synthetic medicines.

This book specially focuses on the herbal medicinal antibiotics and antiviral. All the information given in the book has been very minutely researched and verified by professionals. So if you intend to start living by the cures of our ancestors, we suggest you order this book as soon as possible.

www.ingramcontent.com/pod-product-compliance
Lightning Source LLC
Chambersburg PA
CBHW070241290526
45789CB00004B/1712